PROSTATE ENLARGEMENT UNCOVERED

Insights, Treatments, and Lifestyle Tips for a Healthy Prostate

By

Dr. Andrew Morrison

TABLE OF CONTENTS

CHAPTER SIX

PROSTATE ENLARGEMENT IN THE FUTURE: PERSPECTIVES AND RESEARCH

CONCLUSION

INTRODUCTION

PROSTATE ENLARGEMENT UNCOVERED: *Insights, Treatments, and Lifestyle Tips for a Healthy Prostate* is my most recent book, and I'm pleased to share it with you. This book is intended to be your comprehensive resource if you or a loved one are looking for knowledge and helpful advice on treating prostate enlargement.

I have gathered a wealth of knowledge in this book to assist you in understanding the issue, navigating the various treatment options, and making decisions regarding your prostate health. This book is designed to satisfy your needs, whether you are in the early stages of prostate disease, have just received a diagnosis, or just wish to take preventative measures for a healthy prostate.

Beyond a cursory grasp of the problem, **"PROSTATE ENLARGEMENT UNCOVERED"** explores its root origins, risk factors, and most recent scientific findings. You'll learn useful information about various conventional and alternative treatment modalities as well as useful lifestyle advice that can help to promote prostate health.

The emphasis on empowering you to take charge of your own wellbeing is what distinguishes this book from others. You'll discover practical tips, self-care routines, and guidance on leading a full life despite prostate enlargement throughout the book's pages.

On this enlightening and powerful exploration of prostate enlargement, I cordially welcome you to join me. **'Prostate Enlargement Uncovered'** wants to be your trusted companion, giving you the information and resources you need to make informed decisions and lead a healthy, balanced life, whether you are a patient, caretaker, or healthcare professional.

We appreciate you taking a look at **'Prostate Enlargement Uncovered.'** It will, in my opinion, be a priceless tool for you as you work toward prostate health and wellbeing. Let's take control of our prostate health together and unleash the potential for a happy life.

I'm wishing you the best of luck on your travels.

ABSTRACT

A lot of men experience prostate enlargement, commonly known as benign prostatic hyperplasia (BPH), especially as they get older. In-depth knowledge of prostate enlargement, including its causes, symptoms, techniques of diagnosis, and potential treatments, is the goal of this book. The knowledge provided in this book will enable readers to understand this widespread disorder and make wise decisions about their health.

The urethra, the tube that takes urine from the bladder out of the body, is surrounded by the prostate gland, a little gland about the size of a walnut that is situated right below the bladder. Its primary job is to produce the seminal fluid necessary for sperm nutrition and transportation during ejaculation.

The prostate gland grows normally as men age, and in some situations, it may enlarge. While the precise origin of prostate enlargement is unknown, it is thought to be impacted by hormonal changes, especially a rise in the hormone dihydrotestosterone (DHT), which is a testosterone analogue.

Prostate enlargement symptoms can include:

- ❖ Urge to urinate frequently or immediately
- ❖ Difficulty beginning to urinate
- ❖ Weak urine flow
- ❖ An incomplete bladder emptying
- ❖ After the conclusion of urination, dribbling
- ❖ Struggling to urinate
- ❖ Nocturia (regular nighttime urination)
- ❖ urinary retention (inability to totally empty the bladder)

These signs and symptoms can have an uncomfortable impact on a man's quality of life and interfere with regular activities. The fact that prostate enlargement is a non-cancerous condition and does not raise the risk of getting prostate cancer is crucial to remember.

Typically, a complete medical history, physical examination, and a number of tests are used to diagnose prostate enlargement. A digital rectal examination (DRE), a blood test for prostate-specific antigen (PSA), and occasionally imaging procedures like an ultrasound or a cystoscopy to examine the urinary tract are among the possible testing.

The impact of prostate enlargement on a man's life and the intensity of his symptoms will determine how best to treat him. Typical forms of treatment include:

In moderate circumstances, the doctor may monitor the illness without taking any direct action.

Medications: To assist in relaxing the prostate muscles and reducing its size, physicians may prescribe alpha-blockers and 5-alpha reductase inhibitors.

Procedures with a low risk of complications include laser therapy, prostatic stents, and transurethral resection of the prostate (TURP), among others.

Surgery: Prostate tissue removal surgery may be advised in more severe situations or if other therapies are inadequate.

Monitoring the condition and addressing any potential problems requires regular check-ups and conversations with a healthcare practitioner.

As with any medical condition, it's crucial to speak with a licensed healthcare provider for a precise diagnosis, individualized guidance, and suitable treatment options.

CHAPTER ONE

PROSTATE ENLARGEMENT EXPLAINED

Recap of important points

Early detection and proactive management are crucial.

This book aims to increase knowledge and comprehension of prostate enlargement by examining the causes, symptoms, diagnoses, and available treatments. In order to promote prompt intervention and improved quality of life for those affected, it is essential for both healthcare professionals and patients to stay aware about prostate enlargement.

Benign prostatic hyperplasia (BPH), a condition in which the prostate gland experiences non-cancerous development and expansion, is referred to as prostate enlargement. Men's prostate glands are little, walnut-sized organs that are situated next to the bladder. The urethra, the tube that takes urine from the bladder out of the body, can get compressed as a result of the prostate gland's tendency to enlarge with age. Numerous symptoms and issues related to the urinary system might arise from this growth. Although prostate enlargement is not malignant, if left untreated, it can have a substantial negative influence on a man's quality of life.

Amount and importance of the conditions

BPH, also known as benign prostatic hyperplasia, is more common as people get older. Up to 90% of men in their 70s and 80s and over 50% of men in their 60s are thought to have some degree of prostate enlargement. Men under the age of 40 have a lower prevalence of the illness.

Due to the possible effects it could have on a man's quality of life and general health, prostate enlargement is regarded as a serious condition. Lower urinary tract symptoms (LUTS), also known as lower urinary symptoms (LUS), can be brought on by an enlarged prostate. Urinary hesitancy, poor urine flow, frequent urination (particularly at night), urgency, partial bladder emptying, and the need to strain while urinating are a few examples of these symptoms. Infections, bladder stones, urine retention (the inability to completely empty the bladder), and even kidney damage can result from prostate enlargement if it is not addressed.

It is important to recognize how enlarged prostate affects a man's quality of life. LUTS can interfere with regular sleep cycles, which can result in weariness and decreased productivity during the day. Additionally, it can make people feel embarrassed in front of others and prevent them from taking part in activities that need them to spend a lot of time outside of the bathroom.

To reduce symptoms, avoid problems, and enhance the general wellbeing of those affected by prostate enlargement, early detection, accurate diagnosis, and care are essential. Addressing the incidence and importance of this issue requires regular screening and open dialogue with medical providers.

PROSTATE PHYSIOLOGY AND ANATOMY

An essential part of the male reproductive system is the prostate gland. It is a walnut-sized gland that is situated in front of the rectum, just below the bladder. The ejaculatory ducts, which move semen during ejaculation, and the urethra, the tube that takes urine from the bladder out through the penis, are both encircled by the prostate.

The following main structures make up the prostate's anatomy:

1.**Prostatic Capsule**: A fibrous capsule that surrounds and contains the prostate offers structural support.

2. **Lobes**: The prostate gland's three lobes—the central, transitional, and peripheral—are frequently discussed. The innermost area, known as the central zone, is where the ejaculatory ducts are formed. In cases of benign prostatic hyperplasia (BPH), the transitional zone, which encircles the urethra, is the region most susceptible to growth. The majority of prostate tumours start in the peripheral zone, which is the greatest area.

3.**Zones and Ducts**: Anatomical zones can also be used to classify the prostate. The majority of cases of prostate cancer start in the peripheral zone, which makes up roughly 70% of the gland. The majority of instances of BPH are caused by the transition zone, which encircles the urethra. The ejaculatory ducts are located in the middle zone, which is the smallest area.

4.**Ductal System**: Several ducts in the prostate connect to the prostatic urethra. A milky fluid that is secreted by these ducts makes up a sizable portion of semen. The fluid is abundant in zinc, citric acid, enzymes, and prostate-specific antigen (PSA), which promotes the survival and function of sperm.

The prostate gland's secretory and muscular processes are part of its physiology:

1.**Secretory Function:** The prostate gland produces a milky secretion that aids in the production of semen. This fluid's alkaline nature helps to balance the vagina's acidic environment, improving sperm viability and motility. The prostate produces a protein called prostate-specific antigen (PSA), which aids in the liquefaction of semen following ejaculation.

2.**Muscular Activity:** Smooth muscles in the prostate contract during ejaculation. These contractions aid in the movement of semen into the urethra and ejaculatory ducts.

Hormonal signals, notably androgens like testosterone, have an impact on the prostate gland and its operations. The size and function of the prostate gland can be affected by changes in hormone levels, aging-related changes, and other variables, which can result in diseases such prostate enlargement (BPH) or prostate cancer. Understanding the etiology and treatment of prostate-related illnesses requires knowledge of the anatomy and physiology of the prostate.

CHAPTER TWO

FUNCTION AND STRUCTURE OF THE PROSTATE GLAND

In males, the prostate gland is a tiny, walnut-sized gland that is situated immediately below the bladder. It is a component of the male reproductive system and is essential for the generation and movement of sperm. The prostate gland's anatomy and operation are as follows:

Structure:

1. **Location**: The prostate gland is placed right below the bladder and in front of the rectum. It encircles the urethra, which is the tube that empties the body of urine and sperm.

2. **Size and Shape**: The prostate gland can vary in size and shape from person to person, but on average, it measures around 4 centimeters in diameter and 3 centimeters in height. It is conical in shape, with the apex pointing in the direction of the penis and the base facing the bladder.

3.**Lobes:** There are various lobes that split the prostate gland. The anterior lobe, posterior lobe, and two lateral lobes are the most important divisions.

4.**Histological Structure**: The prostate gland is made up of several tissue types under the microscope. Seminal fluid is created by the glandular tissue, which is made up of glandular cells. The supportive tissue, or stroma, gives the gland its structural integrity.

Function:

1.**Production of Seminal Fluid:** The prostate gland's main job is to create a sizeable amount of the seminal fluid, which supports and carries sperm. About 20–30% of the entire amount of semen is made up of a milky, alkaline secretion produced by the glandular cells in the prostate.

2.**Ejaculation:** During ejaculation, the prostate gland's muscles flex, assisting the seminal fluid's entry into the urethra. After passing via the urethra and the penis, this sperm and seminal fluid mixture leaves the body.

3.**Prostate-Specific Antigen (PSA):** The prostate gland also secretes a molecule known as PSA. The semen is helped to liquefy by the enzyme PSA, which makes it easier for it to flow. PSA blood levels are frequently measured as a screening test for prostate health.

4.**Effect on Urination:** The prostate gland's proximity to the urethra makes it possible for it to have an effect on urination. It is possible for the urethra to get compressed as the prostate gland becomes older (a disease known as benign prostatic hyperplasia, or BPH), which can lead to urinary symptoms like frequent urination, poor urine flow, and trouble starting or ending urination.

It's crucial to remember that the prostate gland is also prone to a number of ailments, including prostatitis (inflammation of the prostate), prostate cancer, and other illnesses that may call for medical treatment. The early detection and treatment of any possible problems can be aided by routine examinations and screenings.

The prostate's function inside the male reproductive system

An essential part of the male reproductive system is the prostate gland. It is a walnut-sized gland that surrounds the urethra, the tube through which urine and semen exit the body, directly below the bladder. The prostate gland is essential to the male reproductive system in a number of ways, including:

1.**Production of Semen:** A large amount of semen is produced by the prostate gland, which secretes a milky fluid. The proteins, enzymes, and nutrients in this fluid support and safeguard sperm cells.

2.**Sperm Activation:** Sperm cells are more easily mobilized and better able to fertilize an egg when they are activated and energized by the prostate gland's secretions.

3.**Production of PSA:** The prostate gland produces PSA, an enzyme that aids in the liquefaction of semen following ejaculation. Sperm migration within the female reproductive system is facilitated by this liquefaction.

4. **Muscle Contraction:** During ejaculation, semen is propelled by the smooth muscles of the prostate gland. These contractions assist in moving the semen out of the penis and via the urethra.

5.**Prostatic Fluid Buffering:** By neutralizing the acidity in the urethra and vaginal tract, prostatic fluid helps to create an environment that is more conducive to sperm survival and motility.

The prostate gland is a key component of the male reproductive system, but it is also susceptible to diseases that can impair its function, including prostatitis (prostate inflammation), benign prostatic hyperplasia (prostate enlargement), and prostate cancer.

For maintaining prostate health and spotting any potential problems early on, routine medical exams and tests are crucial.

CHAPTER THREE

PROSTATE ENLARGEMENT CAUSES

BPH, or benign prostatic hyperplasia, is a disorder that commonly affects elderly men and causes prostate enlargement. Although the precise origin of BPH is not fully understood, many variables are thought to play a role in its occurrence. Here are a few potential reasons:

1.**Age:** Aging is the main factor in prostate hypertrophy. The prostate gland naturally expands in size as men age. The percentage of males who have some degree of prostate enlargement by the age of 40 rises with age.

2. **Hormonal alterations:** Prostate enlargement is thought to be influenced by changes in hormone levels, specifically an increase in levels of the hormone dihydrotestosterone (DHT), which is generated from testosterone. DHT encourages prostate cell expansion, which results in an enlarged prostate.

3.**Family history**: Prostate enlargement appears to have a genetic component. A guy may have an increased risk of acquiring prostate enlargement if his father or sibling have the ailment.

4.**Hormonal imbalances:** Prostate enlargement can be exacerbated by hormonal imbalances, such as a drop in testosterone or an increase in estrogen. However, further research is still needed to determine the precise connection between BPH and hormonal abnormalities.

5. **Chronic inflammation:** BPH development may be correlated with chronic inflammation of the prostate gland. The prostate tissue may enlarge and get larger due to inflammation.

6.**Obesity:** Some data point to an association between obesity and a higher risk of BPH development. Although the exact mechanisms underlying this association are not fully understood, it is thought that obesity may cause hormonal imbalances and chronic inflammation, both of which can result in enlarged prostates.

7.**Lifestyle variables:** Smoking, a poor diet, and a sedentary lifestyle are some lifestyle factors that may raise the risk of prostate enlargement. On the other hand, consistent exercise and a balanced diet may help lower the risk.

While it's crucial to keep in mind that these factors may contribute to prostate enlargement, research into the precise causes and mechanisms of BPH is currently underway. It is advisable to speak with a healthcare provider if you are showing signs of prostate enlargement in order to receive a precise diagnosis and viable treatment choices.

PROSTATE ENLARGEMENT SYMPTOMS AND CLINICAL EFFECTS

As men age, they are more likely to develop prostate enlargement, also known as benign prostatic hyperplasia (BPH). The prostate gland, which surrounds the urethra and is situated directly below the bladder, can gradually grow in size, resulting in a variety of symptoms and clinical implications. Here are some typical signs of prostate enlargement and their clinical implications:

Urinary symptoms: The enlarged prostate can lead to urinary issues like: as it presses against the urethra.

An increased need to urinate more frequently, both during the day and at night (nocturia), may be experienced by men with BPH.

Urgency: There can be an urgent, intense need to urinate, which could occasionally cause leakage or make it difficult to contain urine.

Weak urine flow: Urination may start taking longer to complete and may become weaker or more hesitant.

Men with BPH may find it difficult to begin urinating or to finish emptying their bladders completely.

Dribbling after urination: The flow of urine may persist for a short while after it has stopped.

Urinary tract infections (UTIs): In some circumstances, BPH may make UTIs more likely. Incomplete bladder emptying brought on by obstruction of the urine flow brought on by an enlarged prostate can foster bacterial development.

Bladder stones: Stagnant urine can encourage the development of bladder stones when the bladder does not completely drain owing to BPH. These stones may need to be removed because they can be uncomfortable.

Acute urine retention: BPH can cause acute urinary retention in extreme situations, which prevents the bladder from emptying at all. In order to treat the obstruction in this condition, catheterization is frequently necessary.

Hematuria: Prostate enlargement may result in hematuria, or blood in the urine. Blood can either be seen or only detected through microscopic analysis.

The signs and clinical effects of prostate enlargement can differ from person to person, it's crucial to remember that. While some BPH-afflicted men may only have moderate symptoms, others may struggle with more serious urinary issues. It is advised to speak with a healthcare provider if you have any urinary symptoms or concerns in order to receive an accurate diagnosis and the best course of treatment.

CHAPTER FOUR

TECHNIQUES FOR DIAGNOSING ENLARGED PROSTATE

BPH, or benign prostatic hyperplasia, is another name for the disorder that causes the prostate to expand. To assess prostate enlargement and gauge its severity, a variety of diagnostic techniques are performed. Here are a few typical diagnostic techniques:

A healthcare expert does a digital rectal examination (DRE) by inserting a finger into the rectum while wearing gloves and lubricant to feel the prostate gland's size, shape, and consistency. This examination may reveal an enlarged prostate.

Prostate-Specific Antigen (PSA) Test: PSA, a protein produced by the prostate gland, is measured in the blood by the PSA test. Increased PSA levels can be a sign of prostate cancer or other problems affecting the prostate, like enlargement. However, it's crucial to remember that elevated PSA levels can also result from other causes, so more testing is typically necessary for a conclusive diagnosis.

Transrectal Ultrasound (TRUS): With the help of sound waves and a tiny probe put into the rectum, TRUS uses sound to provide real-time images of the prostate gland. This imaging method aids in determining the prostate's size and identifying any anomalies or indicators of enlargement.

Uroflowmetry: During urination, the volume and flow of urine are measured. An enlarged prostate that is impeding the urine flow may be the cause of a decreased flow rate.

Cystoscopy: To view the prostate and bladder, a thin, flexible tube with a camera (cystoscope) is inserted via the urethra. Direct prostate viewing is possible, making it easier to spot any enlargement or other abnormalities.

Prostate Biopsy: A prostate biopsy may be carried out in some circumstances where prostate cancer is suspected or to rule out other underlying diseases. Small tissue samples are taken from the prostate gland and examined under a microscope.

Additional imaging tests: To evaluate the size and shape of the prostate and rule out other disorders, additional imaging tests may be utilized, such as magnetic resonance imaging (MRI) or computed tomography (CT) scans.

Depending on the healthcare professional, the patient's symptoms, and the preliminary findings, different diagnostic techniques may be employed. A healthcare practitioner should be consulted for a precise diagnosis and a suitable treatment strategy.

PROSTATE ENLARGEMENT GRADE AND STAGE

A frequent issue that commonly affects older men is prostate enlargement. The prostate enlargement grading and staging systems are intended to evaluate the severity and development of the problem. It's crucial to remember that there are many grading and staging systems depending on the particular condition being assessed. The following are the grading and staging systems for benign prostatic hyperplasia (BPH), the most frequent cause of prostate enlargement:

Assessment of BPH:

The International Prostate Symptom Score (IPSS), commonly referred to as the American Urological Association Symptom Index, is frequently used to quantify BPH. This grading scale evaluates the seriousness of BPH-related urine symptoms. It asks about the occurrence and severity of symptoms such weak urine stream, urgency, hesitation, incomplete bladder emptying, and nocturia (getting up in the middle of the night to urinate). Higher ratings indicate more severe symptoms. The scores range from 0 to 35.

A stage of BPH is:

BPH does not have a recognized staging system, unlike cancer. However, the size of the prostate and the level of obstruction brought on by the enlarged prostate may be used by medical specialists to identify the condition's stage. Typical staging techniques include:

Size of Prostate

A digital rectal examination (DRE) or imaging procedures like transrectal ultrasound (TRUS) or magnetic resonance imaging (MRI) can be used to measure the size of the prostate. Larger prostate sizes may indicate more advanced stages of BPH. Prostate size is commonly measured in cubic centimeters (cc) or milliliters (ml).

Obstruction Level:

Tests like uroflowmetry and post-void residual (PVR) urine volume measurement can be performed to assess the degree of obstruction brought on by an enlarged prostate. While PVR gauges the volume of pee still in the bladder after voiding, uroflowmetry gauges the rate at which urine flows during urination. Higher blockage readings could be a sign of advanced BPH.

These grading and staging systems aid medical practitioners in determining the best prostate enlargement management plan and gauging the severity of urine symptoms. It's crucial to speak with a healthcare professional for a thorough assessment and individualized treatment plan.

CHAPTER FIVE

PROSTATE ENLARGEMENT TREATMENT OPTIONS

BPH, also known as benign prostatic hyperplasia (BPH), is a common disorder in elderly men that causes the prostate to expand. Even if it does not pose a life-threatening hazard, it can still result in unwelcome urinary symptoms. Prostate enlargement can be treated in a variety of ways, from noninvasive methods to more invasive surgeries. The following are some popular forms of treatment:

Watchful Waiting: Your doctor may advise a "watchful waiting" strategy if your symptoms are minor and not adversely affecting your quality of life. This entails ongoing observation of your situation without prompt intervention.

Lifestyle Modifications: Some lifestyle adjustments can help manage BPH's minor symptoms. These include consuming fewer fluids before bed, abstaining from coffee and alcohol, and voiding the bladder entirely.

Medications: BPH can be treated with a number of different drugs. These consist of:

Tamsulosin, alfuzosin, and terazosin are examples of medications that relax the muscles in the prostate and bladder, improving urine flow and easing symptoms.

5-Alpha-Reductase Inhibitors: Drugs like finasteride and dutasteride operate by lowering the production of hormones that cause enlargement of the prostate. Over time, these medications can aid in prostate shrinkage and symptom relief.

Alpha-blockers and 5-alpha-reductase inhibitors may be used in combination therapy for some men to get improved symptom relief.

Minimally Invasive techniques: Several minimally invasive techniques might be taken into consideration if drugs are insufficient or well-tolerated.

Transurethral Microwave Thermotherapy (TUMT) employs microwave energy to heat and eliminate extra prostate tissue, hence lessening discomfort related to the urethra.

Transurethral Needle Ablation (TUNA): TUNA is a procedure in which radiofrequency energy is delivered through needles into the prostate to burn away the enlarging tissue.

By using lasers to remove extra prostate tissue, procedures including photoselective vaporization of the prostate (PVP) and holmium laser enucleation of the prostate (HoLEP) can relieve urinary blockage.

Surgery may be required in more severe situations or after all other therapies have failed. Transurethral resection of the prostate (TURP) is the surgical procedure that is most frequently used. Using a resectoscope introduced through the urethra, the obstructive prostate tissue is removed during this surgery.

It's crucial to speak with a medical expert to choose the best course of action for your particular illness because it relies on the intensity of your symptoms, the size of your prostate, your general health, and your preferences.

PROSTATE ENLARGEMENT EDUCATION AND COUNSELLING FOR PATIENTS

There are several crucial topics to discuss when it comes to patient education and counseling on prostate enlargement, commonly known as benign prostatic hyperplasia (BPH). Here is a detailed guide on the subject:

In order to better understand BPH, let's first go through what it is and how it affects the prostate gland. Reiterate that BPH is a non-cancerous disorder in which the prostate gland gradually enlarges, causing urine symptoms such increased frequency, urgency, weak flow, trouble starting or stopping urination, and incomplete bladder emptying.

Risk Factors: Talk about the factors that increase the risk of BPH. The illness is more prevalent in men over 50, making age the biggest risk factor. BPH can also be influenced by a person's family history, hormone imbalances, and specific medical problems (such as obesity and diabetes).

Symptoms: Describe in full the common BPH symptoms. Patients should be advised that the symptoms may affect their quality of life and range in severity. Tell them to get checked out by a doctor if they have any urinary symptoms so that other problems can be ruled out.

Diagnosis: Outline the BPH diagnostic procedure. Mention that it typically entails a thorough evaluation of the patient's medical history, a physical examination (including a digital rectal exam), urine tests to rule out infection, and maybe additional tests like a

PSA blood test or imaging procedures (such as an ultrasound or cystoscopy).

Discuss the many BPH treatment options that are available, which might include everything from lifestyle changes to prescription medications and surgical procedures. Typical strategies include:

In cases of minor symptoms, people may decide to constantly monitor their health without seeking immediate medical attention, particularly if the symptoms have little to no influence on their everyday lives.

Encourage patients to make healthy lifestyle adjustments, such as frequent exercise, maintaining a healthy weight, avoiding coffee and alcohol, and limiting fluid intake before bedtime, as these modifications may help reduce symptoms.

Alpha-blockers (such as tamsulosin, terazosin) and 5-alpha reductase inhibitors (such as finasteride, dutasteride) are two frequent drugs recommended to treat BPH. Explain how the medication works, any possible adverse effects, and the value of routine follow-ups to determine the drug's efficacy.

Transurethral microwave therapy (TUMT), transurethral needle ablation (TUNA), and laser therapies (such as photoselective vaporization of the prostate and holmium laser enucleation of the prostate) are examples of minimally invasive treatments. These techniques seek to reduce the size of the prostate gland to alleviate discomfort.

Surgical Interventions: Talk about possible surgical procedures like laser prostatectomy or transurethral resection of the prostate (TURP). Describe how these treatments entail removing or shrinking the prostate gland in order to relieve urinary problems. Explain any potential dangers, advantages, and the length of each surgery's recuperation period.

Follow-up Care: Stress the value of routine follow-up appointments with a healthcare professional to track the development of symptoms, evaluate the efficacy of therapies, and make any required modifications to the management plan.

Briefly describe any probable side effects of BPH, such as acute urine retention, recurring urinary tract infections, bladder stones, and kidney issues. Explain that if any of these issues develop, immediate medical assistance is essential.

Addressing Concerns: Encourage patients to express any worries they may have about their condition by answering any questions they may have.

CHAPTER SIX

PROSTATE ENLARGEMENT IN THE FUTURE: PERSPECTIVES AND RESEARCH

Benign prostatic hyperplasia (BPH), often known as prostate enlargement, is a frequent ailment among elderly men as of my most recent knowledge update in September 2021. Even if I don't have access to details about specific developments after that time, I can provide you some broad insights and current research directions in the area of prostate enlargement. It's crucial to remember that advances in medical research are continually changing, thus since my previous update, further advancements could have been made.

Research is being concentrated on the creation of fresh, least invasive BPH treatment methods. These methods seek to effectively relieve symptoms while minimizing negative effects and speeding up the healing process. Examples include water vapor therapy (Rezm), prostatic artery embolization (PAE), and laser ablation methods such as holmium laser enucleation of the prostate (HoLEP) and thulium laser enucleation of the prostate (ThuLEP).

Pharmacological therapy: For the treatment of BPH, researchers are looking into novel pharmacological therapy. These include the creation of innovative medications with increased efficacy and fewer adverse effects, as well as combination medicines that focus on several pathways implicated in prostate enlargement.

Molecular targets are being identified as part of ongoing research with the hope of creating more specialized treatments for prostate enlargement. Researchers hope to create therapies that can halt or stop the growth of BPH by studying the underlying processes and pathways.

Biomarkers: Research is being done to find valid biomarkers for BPH. The use of biomarkers in the early detection, diagnosis, and monitoring of prostate enlargement may enable more specialized therapeutic strategies and better patient results.

Regenerative medicine: To regenerate or repair the prostate tissue damaged by BPH, several researchers are investigating regenerative medicine treatments, including as tissue engineering and stem cell therapy. Although this discipline is still developing, it shows promise for potential therapeutic approaches in the future.

Artificial Intelligence and Machine Learning: Prostate health research is a new area in which artificial intelligence (AI) and machine learning techniques are being applied. In order to increase the precision of diagnosis, the choice of treatment, and patient outcomes, AI algorithms can help in the analysis of complicated data sets, such as genetic data and medical imaging.

These are only a few areas of prostate enlargement research and development. It is expected that future advancements in the diagnosis, treatment, and management of this ailment will be made as medical knowledge and technology continue to grow.

CONCLUSION

Males frequently experience prostate enlargement, also known as benign prostatic hyperplasia (BPH), especially as they get older. I can give you an overall assessment of prostate enlargement based on the data up to September 2021.

The prostate gland, which is situated below the bladder and encircles the urethra, enlarges, resulting in prostate enlargement. Although the exact cause of this is unknown, it is thought that aging and hormonal changes, particularly an increase in dihydrotestosterone (DHT), are responsible.

Although the signs and symptoms of prostate enlargement might vary, they frequently involve urinary issues such frequent urination, poor urine flow, difficulty initiating and ending urination, and the perception that the bladder is not completely emptying. A person's quality of life may be greatly impacted by these symptoms.

Although prostate enlargement is typically a benign condition and is not associated with prostate cancer, it is always vital to speak with a medical expert to rule out any underlying conditions. A complete medical history, physical examination, and maybe further tests like a PSA blood test, a urine flow study, or an ultrasound are usually required to diagnose BPH.

The intensity of the symptoms and how they affect daily life will determine the best course of action for treating prostate enlargement. Changes in lifestyle, such as abstaining from caffeine and alcohol and employing "bladder training" methods, can help treat mild to moderate cases. Alpha-blockers and 5-alpha reductase inhibitors are two drugs that can be used to treat symptoms and shrink the prostate. Laser surgery or transurethral resection of the prostate (TURP) may be advised in more serious situations.

It is important to note that medical research and developments are continuing, and that since my knowledge cut-off, new therapeutic alternatives or improvements to existing medications may have surfaced. Therefore, in order to receive the most current information and tailored guidance regarding prostate enlargement, it is crucial to speak with a healthcare professional.

www.ingramcontent.com/pod-product-compliance
Lightning Source LLC
Chambersburg PA
CBHW070231260726
48658CB00006BA/2281